3-Day Energizing
& Cleansing Detox

For Spring or Summer

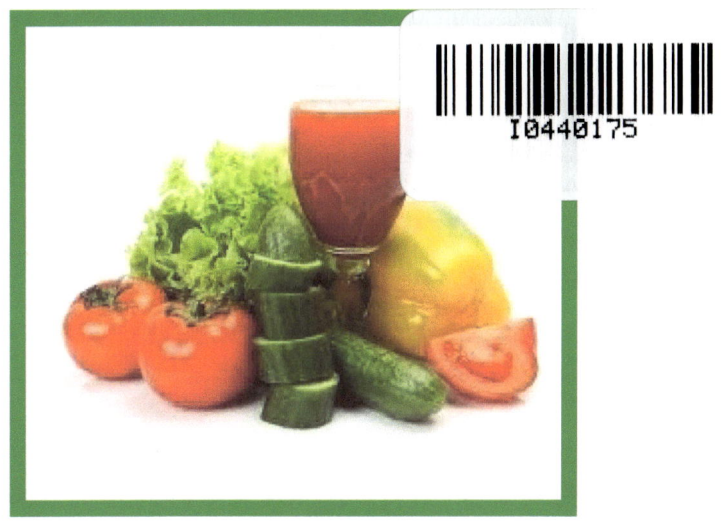

By

Dr. Kathleen B. Oden
Certified Health Minister

Create Anewu Health Ministry

3-DAY ENERGIZING & CLEANSING DETOX

Our bodies are always in a state of detoxing by... Coughing, sneezing, "going" to the bathroom... Ears running or nose dripping!*

It is all detoxing! God made our bodies to naturally "detox" when it needs to get rid of anything that is poison, or waste, or just should not be in the "body."

The body will naturally eject and or reject, anything that needs to go out, of the body.

And if it can't, it's because none of the above* are working properly. Then comes sickness... high blood pressure, diabetes, arthritis, cancer...etc.

3-DAY ENERGIZING & CLEANSING DETOX

CREATE ANEWU 8 to 8 DETOX SCHEDULE

8AM	**Time to rise & energize!**
9AM	**Breakfast Smoothie Time!**
10AM	**Time to Hydrate!**
11AM	**Brunch-a-Soup Time!**
12PM	**Lunch Time Salad!**
1PM	**Afternoon Snack Time!**
2PM	**Time to Juice it up!**
3PM	**Hydrate Time!**
4PM	**Dinner Time Salad!**
5PM	**Time for a Souper Dinner!**
6PM	**Evening Snack Time!**
7PM	**Fruity Smoothie Time!**
8PM	**Good Night Tea Time!**

SHOPPING LIST

6 - lemons
6 - large pieces of raw ginger root
1 - bottle of lemon essential oil
1 - bottle of ginger essential oil
1 - bottle of lavender essential oil
9 - 16 oz. bottles of water
9 - large beef tomatoes
1 - large bag carrots
9 - roma tomatoes
3 - bunch spinach
3 - head romaine lettuce
1 - bottle Bragg's Apple Cider Vinegar
1 - bottle raw olive oil
12 - large apples
3 - large pears
1 - bag frozen strawberries
1 - bag frozen blue berries
1 - bag frozen mango
1 - box chamomile tea

Honey
Sea salt
Garlic Powder

WHEN TO DETOX

Our bodies should be detoxed at the most once a month, if you HAVE NOT, been eating healthy.

However, if you have been eating healthy for at least 1 year, then you only need to detox 3-4 times a year, to keep your body up to par and cleansed!

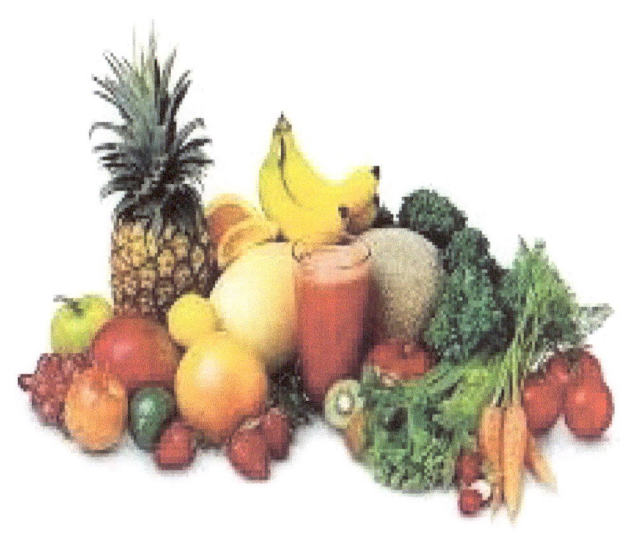

SAMPLE DETOX PLAN

This 3 day energizing & cleansing detox is a sample plan. There are many ways to detox and many ways to prepare your body to detox.

Please feel free to tweak this plan to fit your schedule and lifestyle for example...

EAT MORE VEGGIES & FRUITS

EAT EVERY 2 HOURS

EAT FROM 8AM TO 8PM

DRINK MORE WATER

DRINK GREEN TEA

DRINK MORE SMOOTHIES

DETOX 3-DAY PREP

3 days before you start this detox, start eating light. If you eat a lot of meat, try eating no meat or less meat, for 3 days, before the detox.

Also, 3 days before the detox, drink at least 3-4 10 oz. Bottles of water every day.

WARNING!

CLEAR YOUR SCHEDULE AND BE PREPARE TO STAY AT HOME! THIS IS A CLEANSING DETOX, WHICH MEANS... LOTS OF GOING TO THE BATHROOM!

Don't procrastinate, make a plan. It is better to make a plan so that you will be prepared.

Don't procrastinate, make a plan!

DISCLAIMER

I am not and do not claim to be a medical doctor or a nutritionist.

Please consult with your doctor before doing this or any detox program.

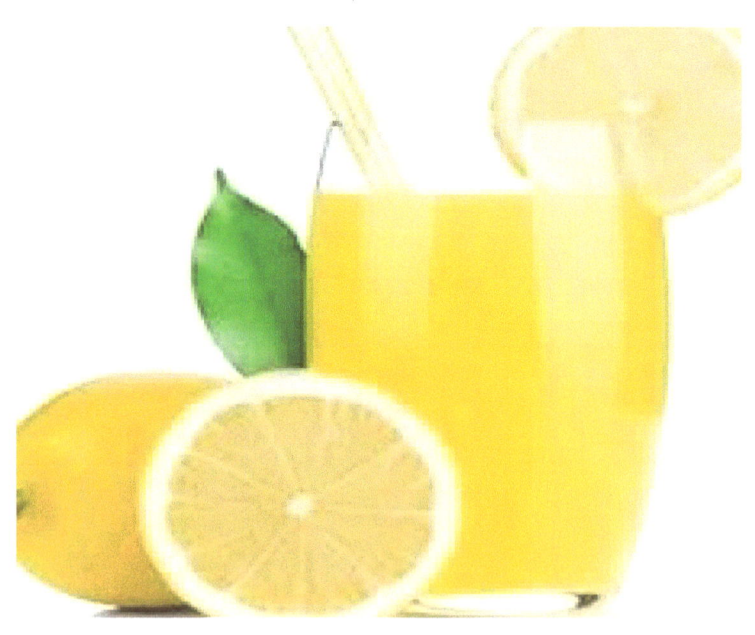

MORNING

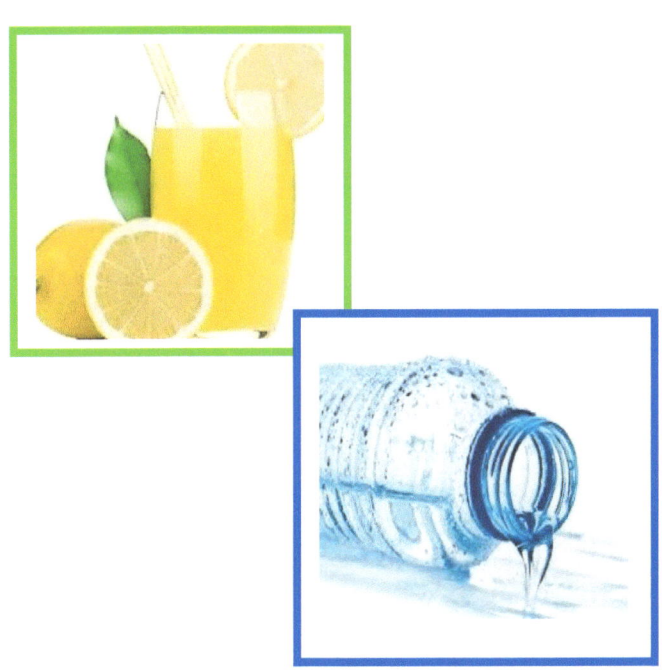

SCHEDULE

Time to rise & energize!

LEMON GINGER DRINK

1 - lemon
1 - drop of lemon essential oil
1 - piece of raw ginger root
1 - drop of ginger essential oil

Pour 8 ozs. of water in a glass.

Extract juice from lemon and add to water. Add essential oils.

Grate a handful of ginger.

Squeeze ginger over glass to add ginger juice.

Stir and enjoy!

9AM

Breakfast Smoothie Time!

PEPPERMINT SMOOTHIE

1 - half a bunch spinach
1 - large apple (remove core)
1 - pear (remove core)
1 - drop peppermint essential oil
1 - 10 oz. of bottled of water

Remove core from apple & pear.

Blend all ingredients in blender.

Enjoy!

10AM

Time to Hydrate!

<u>DRINK WATER</u>

ONE
16 oz.

BOTTLE

OF

WATER

DRINK COLD OR ROOM
TEMPERATURE

11AM

Brunch-a-Soup Time!

<u>TOMATO & CARROT SOUP</u>

1 - large beef tomato
1 - large carrot
8 oz. Of bottled water

Blend all ingredients in blender.

Season with sea salt &
1 tsp. of honey - (optional)
& dash of garlic powder

May be eaten cold or heated for
1 min. or less to preserve
Enzymes.   Sprinkle   shredded
spinach on top.

Enjoy!

AFTERNOON

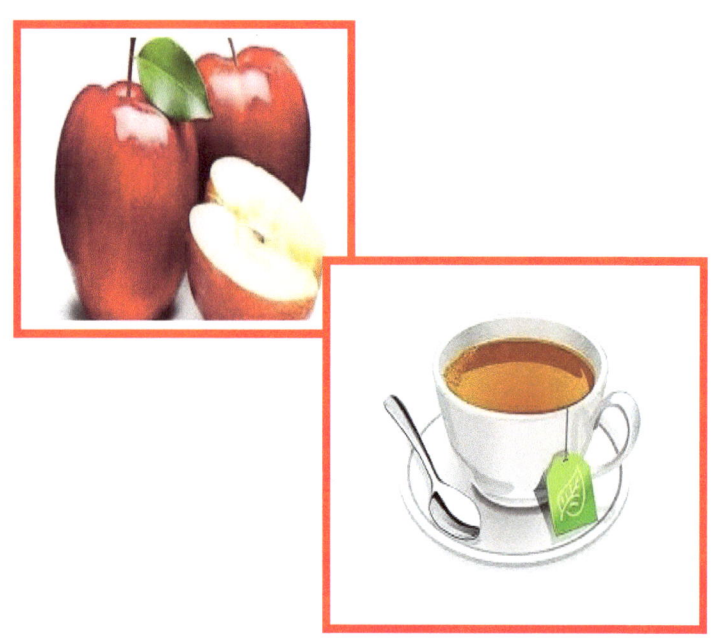

SCHEDULE

12PM

Lunch Time Salad!

HEALTHY GREEN SALAD

2 - cups romaine lettuce
half a bunch spinach
1 - roma tomato
1 - TBS olive oil
1 - TBS apple cider vinegar
1 - TBS honey (optional)
1 - 16 oz. bottle of water

Tear or cut up lettuce and spinach into a salad bowl. Dice tomato and add to bowl.

Pour olive oil and apple cider vinegar in a container and stir or shake to combine ingredients. Pour over salad. Stir salad.

Eat your salad!
Drink your water!

1PM

Afternoon Snack Time!

1 BIG RED JUICY APPLE

CORE THE APPLE

AND CUT INTO

PIECES

OR

JUST EAT IT!

**Do not peel it!
The vitamins are in the skin!**

2PM

Time to Juice it up!

LEMON GINGER DRINK

1 - lemon
1 - drop of lemon essential oil
1 - piece of raw ginger root
1 - drop of ginger essential oil

Pour 8 ozs. of water in a glass.

Extract juice from lemon and add to water. Add essential oils.

Grate a handful of ginger.

Squeeze ginger over glass to add ginger juice.

Stir and enjoy!

3PM

Time to Hydrate!

DRINK WATER

**ONE
16 oz.**

BOTTLE

OF

WATER

**DRINK COLD OR ROOM
TEMPERATURE**

EVENING

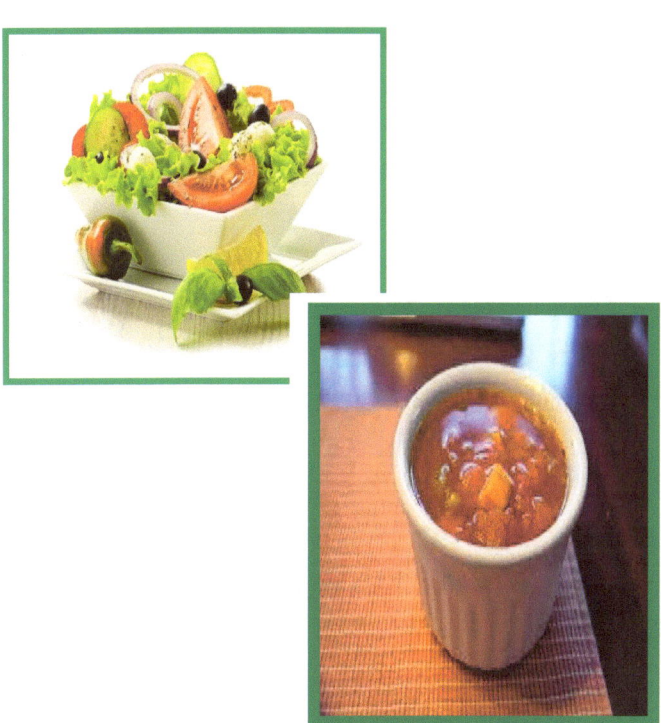

SCHEDULE

4PM

Dinner Time Salad!

HEALTHY GREEN SALAD

2 - cups romaine lettuce
half a bunch spinach
1 - roma tomato
1 - TBS olive oil
1 - TBS apple cider vinegar
1 - TBS honey (optional)
1 - 16 oz. bottle of water

Tear or cut up lettuce and spinach into a salad bowl. Dice tomato and add to bowl.

Pour olive oil and apple cider vinegar in a container and stir or shake to combine ingredients. Pour over salad. Stir salad.

Eat your salad!
Drink your water!

5PM

Time for a Souper Dinner!

<u>TOMATO & CARROT SOUP</u>

1 - large beef tomato
1 - large carrot
8 oz. Of bottled water

Blend all ingredients in blender.

Season with sea salt &
1 tsp. of honey - (optional)
& dash of garlic powder

May be eaten cold or heated for
1 min. or less to preserve
enzymes.   Sprinkle   shredded
spinach on top.

Enjoy!

6PM

Evening Snack Time!

1 BIG RED JUICY APPLE

CORE THE APPLE

AND CUT INTO

PIECES

OR

JUST EAT IT!

Do not peel it!
The vitamins are in the skin!

7PM

Fruity Smoothie Time!

<u>BERRY SWEET SMOOTHIE</u>

Half cup strawberries

1 cup blue berries

Half cup mango

2 - cups ice

16 oz. cold water

Blend all ingredients in blender.

Enjoy!

Good Night Tea Time!

<u>LAVENDER CHAMOMILE TEA</u>

8 - oz. boiled bottled water

2 - chamomile tea bags

1-2 drop lavender essential oil

1 TBS honey (optional)

Pour water into a cup. Let tea bags sit in hot water at least 2 minutes.

Add lavender. Stir, inhale the lavender as you sip your tea.

**Enjoy your tea!
Enjoy your sleep!   zzzzzzz!**

3 JOHN 1:2

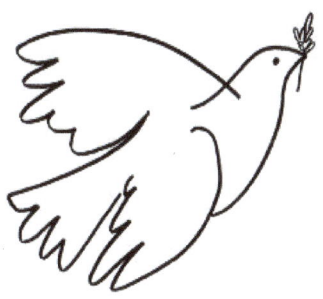

Beloved,
I wish above all things
that thou mayest prosper
and be in health,
even as thy soul prospereth.

Dr. Kathleen B. Oden

Dr. Kathleen B. Oden has been a member of God's House of Refuge Church & School of Evangelism since 1994 and is currently the Church Administrator, Bible teacher and missionary.

She has a Doctorate degree in Christian Theology and she is a Certified Health Minister and Certified Essential Oil Coach.

Dr. Oden hosts healthy living seminars and she also does private health coaching through her ministry, Create AnewU Health Ministry.

She has published over 20 through AMAZON.COM. Dr. Oden is currently working on several new books.

WEBSITE:
createanewuhealthministry.com

EMAIL:
createanewu@consultant.com